Reflexology Made Easy for Seniors

A Comprehensive Handbook to Hand and Foot Reflexology Simplified for Seniors to Deal with Stress, Body Pains and Improve Your Overall Health

Introduction

As years go by, you might quickly discover that your body does not function as well as it used to – which is quite normal. Also, some of the routine activities you enjoyed engaging in may feel more strenuous due to complications related to advancing age.

However, the functional changes in your body do not necessarily have to affect your quality of life, slow you down, or keep you away from the activities you loved in the past.

But how? You may wonder.

That is where reflexology comes into play.

Reflexology is a non-invasive alternative or complementary treatment that revolves around maintenance therapy, preventive care, and pain management, which can be applied to numerous conditions associated with aging. This therapy entails applying gentle pressure to specific points along your hands and feet to assist you in feeling better. Also referred to as zone therapy, reflexology has also been shown to relieve stress and improve your body's overall functioning.

Reflexology falls in the same category as other closely related therapies that promote your overall well-being, such as massage, reiki, chiropractic, and homeopathy. Actually, it slightly resembles massage, but the two are quite different despite sharing some similarities.

Although the exact origins of reflexology remain unknown, the therapy was practiced thousands of years ago in Ancient Egypt and China, according to archeological and historical evidence. For example, an ancient Egyptian papyrus, a document used at the time and dates as far back as 2500 BC, was found to have illustrations of Egyptian medical practitioners performing hand and foot treatments to patients. Stone carvings in India, Japan, Greece, and China depicting ancient practices of healing feet have also been discovered over the years by historians.

Contemporary researchers have also played their part by undertaking studies in an attempt to debunk reflexology, unravel how it works, identify its benefits, and establish its effectiveness. Most scientists agree that when practiced as a holistic approach to complement mainstream forms of treatment, as opposed to curative therapy, seniors can reap numerous benefits from reflexology. These include stress alleviation, pain relief, improved circulation, and enhanced mobility – issues that tend to prevent older adults from living life to the fullest.

If you have always had the desire to try out reflexology but have not had sufficient information to help you make an informed decision, you are in the right place. Hopefully, by the time you turn the last page, you should be armed with the relevant facts that will enable you to decide if reflexology is the solution to your pain points and establish if you are a suitable candidate for this therapy.

But just like any other complementary treatment or wellness practice, **consulting your physician before beginning reflexology is highly recommended**, especially if you are recovering from surgery on any part of your hands or feet. This move serves to ensure that any alternative therapy you may choose to experiment with does not derail or interfere with your recovery process.

However, reflexology is considered relatively safe, and you, too, can enjoy its immense benefits that have the potential to improve your quality of life and physical and mental health.

PS: I'd like your feedback. If you are happy with this book, please leave a review on Amazon.

Please leave a review for this book on Amazon by visiting the page below:

https://amzn.to/2VMR5qr

Table of Contents

Introduction ___ 2

Chapter 1: How Reflexology Works ___ 9

Reflexology Theories ___ 10

Does Reflexology Actually Work? ___ 13

Chapter 2: Proven Benefits of Reflexology and Possible Risks ___ 17

The Benefits ___ 17

Side-Effects and Potential Risks of Reflexology ___ 21

Chapter 3: Foot and Hand Mapping in Reflexology ___ 27

Feet Mapping: A Reflection of Your Body ___ 29

Hand Mapping in Reflexology ___ 34

Cross-Reflexes ___ 37

Chapter 4: Reading and Interpreting Feet in Reflexology ___ 41

Physical Examination _____ 42

Importance of Healthy Feet in Reflexology ____ 44

What Your Feet Reveal _____ 46

What Your Nails Reveal in Reflexology _____ 53

What Are You Eating? _____ 54

Basic Nail Care _____ 56

Chapter 5: How A Reflexology Session Looks Like and What to Expect _____ 58

Personal Preps _____ 59

Setting the Right Mood _____ 62

The Main Event _____ 64

Follow-up Sessions _____ 67

How Should You Expect to Feel After a Reflexology Session? _____ 69

The Healing Crisis Reaction _____ 71

Chapter 6: Emotional and Mental Health Implications of Reflexology _____ 73

How Does Reflexology Boost Emotional and Mental Health? _____ 79

Parting Shot _____ **88**

Chapter 1: How Reflexology Works

As mentioned earlier, reflexology is a wellness practice that encompasses applying gentle pressure to your hands, feet, and sometimes ears. Reflexology is guided by the theory that each of your body parts is linked to specific body systems and organs. By stimulating your reflex points using varying amounts of pressure, **the main objective is to enhance your body's natural healing capabilities, eradicate discomfort, reduce stress and anxiety, and improve mobility.**

Specialists trained to practice this therapy are called reflexologists.

Note: No scientific evidence proves beyond doubt that reflexology prevents or cures any type of ailment. This is why it is considered a form of complementary therapy, which means it is supposed to be used alongside conventional medical care – not as a substitute. However, some studies[1]

---

[1] https://doi.org/10.1155/2014/502123

have shown that reflexology can alleviate certain symptoms[2], such as anxiety and pain. For example, in the case of arthritis, while reflexology may not cure the ailment, it can relieve the joints' inflammation and ease the stiffness associated with the condition.

Although the results of research on the treatment have been mixed, some studies offer a more promising outlook, which makes reflexology a therapy worth trying out.

Reflexology Theories

- **The Chinese Theory**

Reflexology borrows heavily from an old Chinese belief known as *'qi'* (pronounced as *'chee'*), which loosely translates to your *'vital energy.'* This theory argues that everybody possesses qi, which flows through them.

For example, when you feel stressed, your body is blocking qi. In such a scenario, your body experiences an imbalance, which can lead to illness. This is where reflexology can be

---

[2] https://www.cancerresearchuk.org/about-cancer/cancer-in-general/treatment/complementary-alternative-therapies/individual-therapies/reflexology?

applied to ensure your qi continues flowing uninterrupted – ultimately maintaining your body's balance and staving off diseases.

According to Chinese treatment, various parts of the body correspond to a variety of pressure points in your body. As such, reflexologists are guided by maps that point out these matching areas in your hands, feet, and ears. This is how reflexologists establish where to apply pressure, and as a result, their touch directs the energy flowing in your body in order to reach the body part, organ, or system that needs healing.

- **The Western Theory**

In the late 19th Century, British scientists discovered that a complex web of nerves connects your internal organs and skin. Additionally, the scientists discovered that the entire nervous system can adjust to external influences – including touch. This means the touch of a reflexologist has the ability to calm your central nervous system, inducing relaxation among a host of other benefits similar to those offered by a massage. This is also referred to as the Zone theory.

- **Other Theories**

✓ Another theory states that reflexology aids in offsetting how your brain registers pain. When gentle pressure is applied to your feet, the relaxing sensation may improve your mood and curb stress. This may cause you to be less inclined to perceive pain as deeply.

✓ Other scientists trust that your brain perceives pain or discomfort as subjective. At times, your brain may respond to pain, while in other instances, pain could be a response to mental or emotional distress elicited by your brain. Therefore, courtesy of a calming touch, reflexology may have the ability to reduce anxiety and fatigue and provide comfort and reassurance.

Does Reflexology Actually Work?

Most of the evidence that supports the effectiveness of reflexology is not conclusive, as mentioned earlier. This is because a huge chunk of it stems from anecdotal evidence (testimonies from people who claim the therapy works) and unreliable, flawed research studies (which use poorly controlled methodologies or small sample sizes). Therefore, more studies in reflexology are still needed.

Regardless, many people, including seniors, tend to feel much better after a reflexology session, which has led to additional theories about why the therapy appears effective.

Factors that may contribute to this positive outcome, and [backed by studies](https://doi.org/10.1016/j.ctcp.2022.101606)[3], include:

---

[3] https://doi.org/10.1016/j.ctcp.2022.101606

- **Ambiance and Environmental Considerations:** During therapy sessions, reflexologists usually use scents, cool music, and soft lighting, which assists in reducing stress and promoting relaxation.

- **Physical Touch:** Studies have shown that a human touch can facilitate healing and provide comfort. Reflexology involves the manipulation of soft tissue, massaging, and stroking.

- **The Placebo Effect:** There is a possibility that having a strong expectation of a positive outcome through suggestion can eventually result in the desired outcome being achieved. This does not imply that the positive outcome is imagined; it only means the positive results may not necessarily be credited to reflexology alone – other factors may have contributed or merged to produce the positive outcome.

- **Reflexologist Support:** Most sessions are conducted as you lie face up, which enables you to talk to your reflexologist and share your worries, concerns, and fears, work through personal challenges you may be facing, or gain clarity on a nagging issue. This psychological support and your body's relaxation response may be attributed to your improved health and overall well-being.

As long as reflexology does not in any way impede standard medical care, or unless you have a condition the therapy may exacerbate, there should be no harm in trying it out. But to be sure, seek medical advice.

Chapter 2: Proven Benefits of Reflexology and Possible Risks

The Benefits

I believe I have mentioned some of the benefits of reflexology in passing, but let us go into a bit of detail in this chapter. Some of the primary benefits reflexology therapy can offer you include:

- **Reduce Anxiety**

A small study[4] observed the effects of a single 30-minute foot reflexology session on lung and breast cancer patients. The results showed recipients of the therapy reported lower levels of anxiety compared to the participants who did not undergo reflexology treatment.

Another slightly larger study[5] was done on patients undergoing heart surgery, where they were offered 20-minute foot reflexology sessions once a day for four consecutive days. The researchers found that those who received therapy had significantly lower levels of anxiety as opposed to the group that did not.

---

[4] https://www.ncbi.nlm.nih.gov/pubmed/10660924
[5] https://www.sciencedirect.com/science/article/pii/S1744388113000753

- **Provide Pain Relief**

A [study][6] conducted by the National Cancer Institute examined the effects of reflexology on 240 women with breast cancer at an advanced stage. At the time, they were all receiving different forms of treatment – like chemotherapy. The results indicated that reflexology significantly reduced some of their symptoms, such as shortness of breath and pain.

- **Improve Blood Circulation**

Reflexology stimulates blood flow, which, in turn, enhances circulation. Healthy circulation is crucial for maintaining the functions of your cardiovascular system. Consequently, this reduces the risk of blood clots and related complications such as headaches and migraines. For example, when pressure is applied to specific reflex points, it increases blood flow to your brain, which, in turn, reduces migraines and headaches.

When your blood circulation improves, your bladder's functions are enhanced, and your risk of developing urinary tract issues is reduced considerably. This is because you can effectively eliminate unwanted foreign substances and toxins

---

[6] https://www.ncbi.nlm.nih.gov/pmc/articles/PMC3137428/

from your body, which shields you from complications that can develop from a compromised urinary system.

- **Enhance Mobility**

Joint stiffness and mobility issues can affect your quality of life by limiting your activities and movements. Reflexology sessions have the ability to relax your muscles, which significantly improves your mobility.

In a single reflexology session, more than 7,000 nerve endings are stimulated, increasing their capacity to function. This promotes flexibility by releasing muscular tension, responsible for stiffness, pain, and muscle weakness.

- **Combat Insomnia**

It is common for seniors to experience erratic sleep patterns. Due to reflexology's soothing and relaxing effects, your sleep quality improves, leading to more restful nights. When reflex areas in your feet are stimulated by therapy, neural pathways are unblocked, which relaxes your body and calms your mind, leading to better sleep quality.

Once your body and mind are relaxed, the treatment can help you reset your health and normal Circadian rhythm (sleep pattern), which enables you to sleep better at night. In addition, if you are suffering from an underlying condition that interrupts your sleep, like pain and muscle aches, reflexology assists in alleviating acute pain and triggering your body's natural healing response.

- **Improve Mental Health**

Reflexology can promote relaxation and a general sense of well-being, which can result in improved emotional stability, moods, and mental health. This is achieved by stimulating your lymphatic and nervous systems, which then encourages your brain to release feel-good hormones called endorphins. As a result, stress and any other mental condition present are tackled by your body's natural coping mechanism.

The ability of reflexology to improve circulation also supplies your brain with sufficient oxygen. This can lead to improved concentration, focus, and sharper cognitive function. Therefore, if your memory seems to be fading, your mind feels foggy, or you are unable to concentrate on a task for long periods, reflexology could provide the much-needed mental boost you require.

When your mental health improves, it is bound to make you feel confident about yourself, which translates to developing a more positive attitude towards life. This could also result in improved relationships and overall life satisfaction.

Reflexology is also a low-risk therapy that can be combined with other forms of treatment without experiencing any significant challenges.

Side-Effects and Potential Risks of Reflexology

A few reports have emerged in the past concerning reflexology. However, the aftereffects are usually mild and tend to disappear shortly after a session. Some of the most notable side effects include:

- Tenderness on the feet

- Increased bathroom visits

- Emotional sensitivity

- Lightheadedness

In case symptoms persist, which is rare, bring them to the attention of your reflexologist or medical care provider.

Additionally, reflexology may not be advisable if you have some pre-existing medical conditions. This is why consulting your physician before embarking on reflexology cannot be emphasized enough. Also, inform your reflexologist beforehand if you have any medical conditions, are undergoing any treatments, or are under any prescribed medication.

Note: In case you have the below health conditions, reflexology may not be appropriate for you:

- Gout
- Feet fungal infections, such as athlete's foot
- Feet blood circulation problems
- Low platelet count, which leads to bruising and bleeding more easily than normal
- Foot ulcers
- Blood clots or inflammation in your leg veins
- Epilepsy
- Thyroid issues
- Open wounds on your hands or feet

Although it may still be possible to undergo reflexology even with the conditions mentioned above, a few precautions may be necessary to put in place to avoid any adverse effects. Also, if your feet have issues, reflexology can always be performed on your hands, and vice versa.

Exercising due diligence when choosing your reflexologist is equally essential. Therefore, **ensure that your therapist is qualified and adequately trained**. You can inquire about where they received their training and ask for evidence to show they are registered with credible professional bodies, like the Association of Reflexologists.

Also, look out for any red flags. For example, a qualified reflexologist should not:

- Claim to be able to cure any ailment or condition

- Purport or attempt to diagnose medical conditions

- Treat specific conditions

- Prescribe medication

- Ask you to undress

- Encourage you to stop taking prescribed medication or try to overrule your physician's recommendations or treatment plans.

- Work against traditional medicine

If you feel uncomfortable for any reason whatsoever, you have every right to stop the session immediately, cancel future appointments, and terminate the services of the reflexologist in question.

You can begin your search for a qualified reflexologist online on industry sites like **the American Reflexology Certification Board**[7] or **Complementary and Natural Healthcare Council**[8]. Here, you will find registered, accredited reflexologists who are well-trained, experienced, and professional – an excellent place to find the right reflexologist close to your area.

Reflexology is all about bringing harmony, a sense of well-being, and balance to your body. With advancing age, sometimes you may feel *'out of sorts."* As such, your body requires equilibrium for it to continue working normally. Even taking a light reflexology session can help you feel grounded.

---

[7] https://arcb.net/
[8] https://www.cnhc.org.uk/

A question that usually pops up is how long reflexology sessions take to produce tangible results. This is almost impossible to tell. However, every journey begins with one tiny step. What is evident is that your decision to commit to reflexology is the important first step in the right direction.

Chapter 3: Foot and Hand Mapping in Reflexology

As we have already discovered, reflexology is therapeutic, relaxing, and non-invasive and can trigger your entire body's healing mechanisms. It also counts as one of the most intelligent forms of therapy; once you understand how it works, you can easily identify areas of your body that are not functioning as expected.

As mentioned earlier, your hands and feet are mapped to represent different reflexes of organs and systems in your body. For example, a section of your big toe serves as your head's reflex point, and when suffering from a headache or migraine, this is the area where your reflexologist will apply gentle pressure. On the other hand, the spinal reflex is located along the inside edge of your foot, also known as the medial aspect – terms and positions you will get acquainted with shortly.

Another important point worth noting is that your left hand and foot represent the body organs and systems found on the left side, while your right foot and hand map out the right side of your body. All vital organs and body parts have corresponding reflex points on your feet.

It is essential to learn the relationship between the reflexes on your feet/hands and the body parts and organs they correspond to; the tool to assist you in achieving this is through mastering reflexology maps. Apart from mapping lessons, understanding the maps can also enable you to conduct reflexology sessions on yourself – or assist someone else in a situation.

The original reflexology maps were designed by **Eunice Ingham**, who is also fondly christened as the *'mother of reflexology.'* The maps utilized anecdotal data acquired in the course of her reflexology work. Since the maps are not an anatomical representation of the human body, you may come across other maps that differ slightly from the original, which is normal. However, throughout this book, we will use Ingham's groundbreaking maps.

A quick tip: The easiest, fastest, and most practical way to grasp the reflexes in your limbs and match them to their respective body organs and systems is to use your feet and hands as a reference point.

Feet Mapping: A Reflection of Your Body

All body organs and parts are typically arranged in relatively the same order across different reflexology charts. Across the entire foot, you will find guidelines that help you associate specific areas of your body with specific reflex points on your feet. For example, your respiratory organs can be found between your feet' shoulder and diaphragm line, and so on.

The feet maps will also be illustrated from various views, angles, or *'aspects,'* as they will be referred to in this book. The aspects of your feet are divided as follows:

- **Plantar aspect** – this is a view of your foot's underside or sole, the part that is normally in contact with the ground

- **Dorsal aspect** – this is a bird's eye view of your foot or the angle you see it when you look down

- **Medial aspect** – represents the inner edge of your foot, which runs from your big toe to your heel

- **Lateral aspect** – refers to the outer edge of your foot, running from your small toe to your heel

Let's discuss each of these aspects.

1. Plantar Aspect

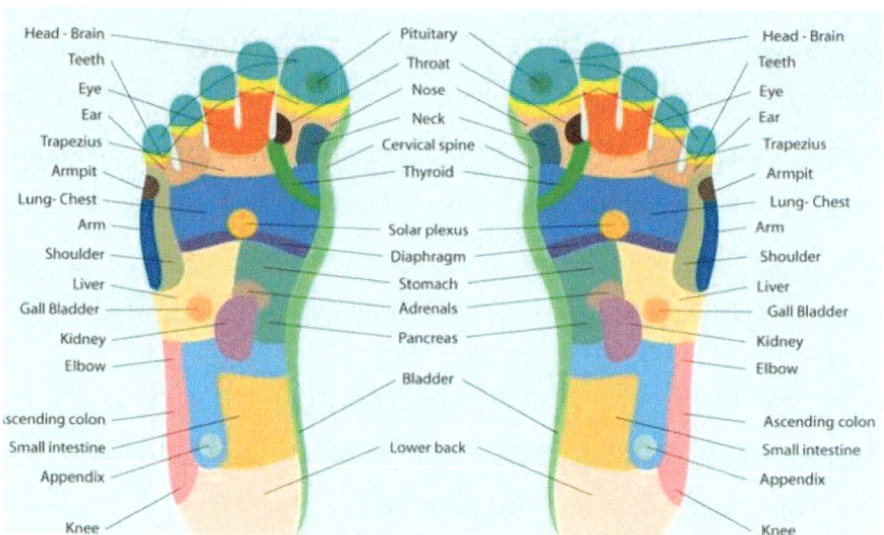

According to Ingham's map, the following are the main parts of the plantar aspect:

✓ **The shoulder line:** This is the area below the bases of both sets of toes. The reflex points of *your head, jaw, ears, eyes, neck, throat, and shoulders* are located just above the shoulder line.

✓ **The diaphragm line** represents the section located under the base of your metatarsals. The area between your shoulder and diaphragm line holds the reflexes of *your gall bladder, pancreas, lungs, hiatus hernia, esophagus, and thyroid.*

- ✓ **Ligament line** – these are the only reflex points that run from top to bottom on your feet – instead of across.

Plantar Foot Map

The plantar foot map illustrates the underside or sole of your feet, which steps on the ground. In reflexology, this is the part of your foot that hosts most of the reflexes, ranging from ***the brain at the tip of your big toe to the sciatic area on your heel.***

2. Dorsal Foot Map

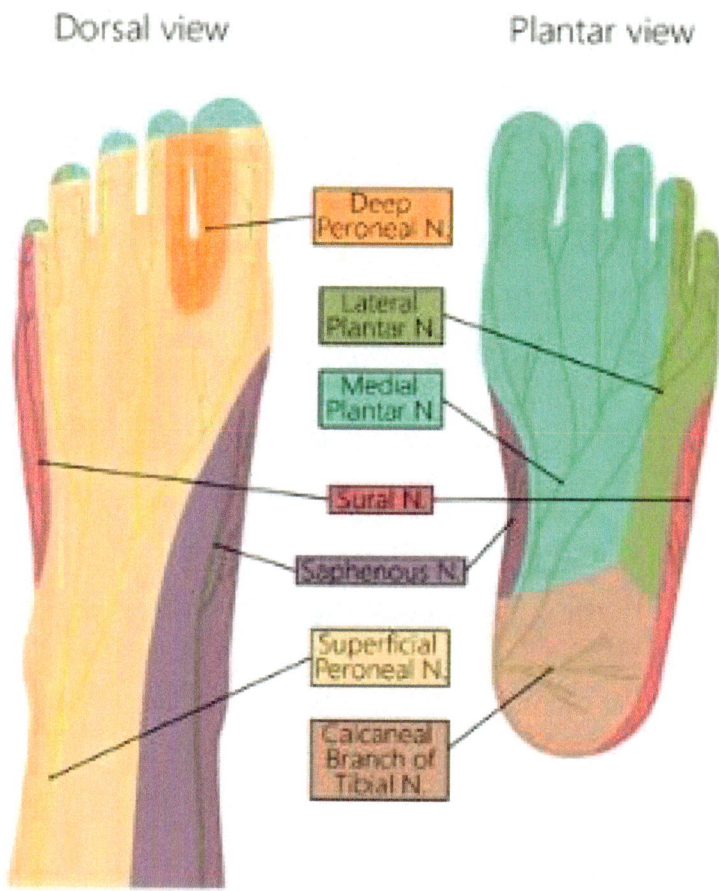

The dorsal map is a representation of the aerial view of your feet and **contains the reflexes of your upper**

lymphatics, throat, jaw, breast, shoulder, and teeth.

3. Median and Lateral Foot Maps

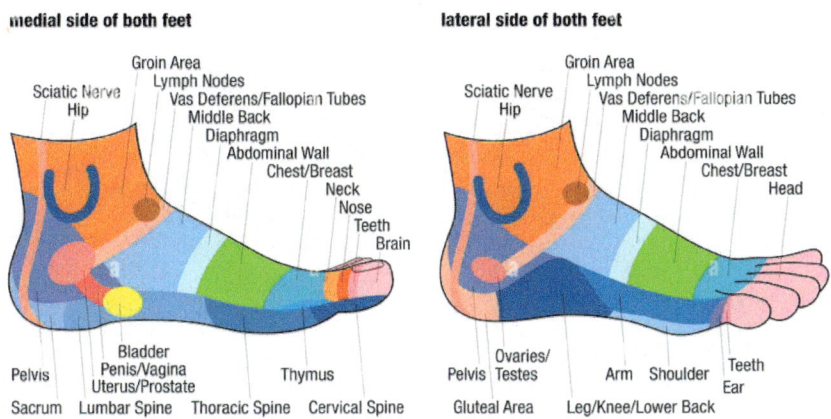

The meridian area is the inner edge of your foot, which runs from the big toe to your heel. Reflexes for *the prostate gland in men, uterus in women, and lumbar, thoracic, and cervical vertebrae* can be found here.

The lateral section is the outer edge of your foot, illustrated in the map above, which extends from your small toe all the way to the heel. The reflex points in this area include *the testes in men and the ovaries in women, as well as the sacrum, hip, knee, shoulder, and elbow.*

Hand Mapping in Reflexology

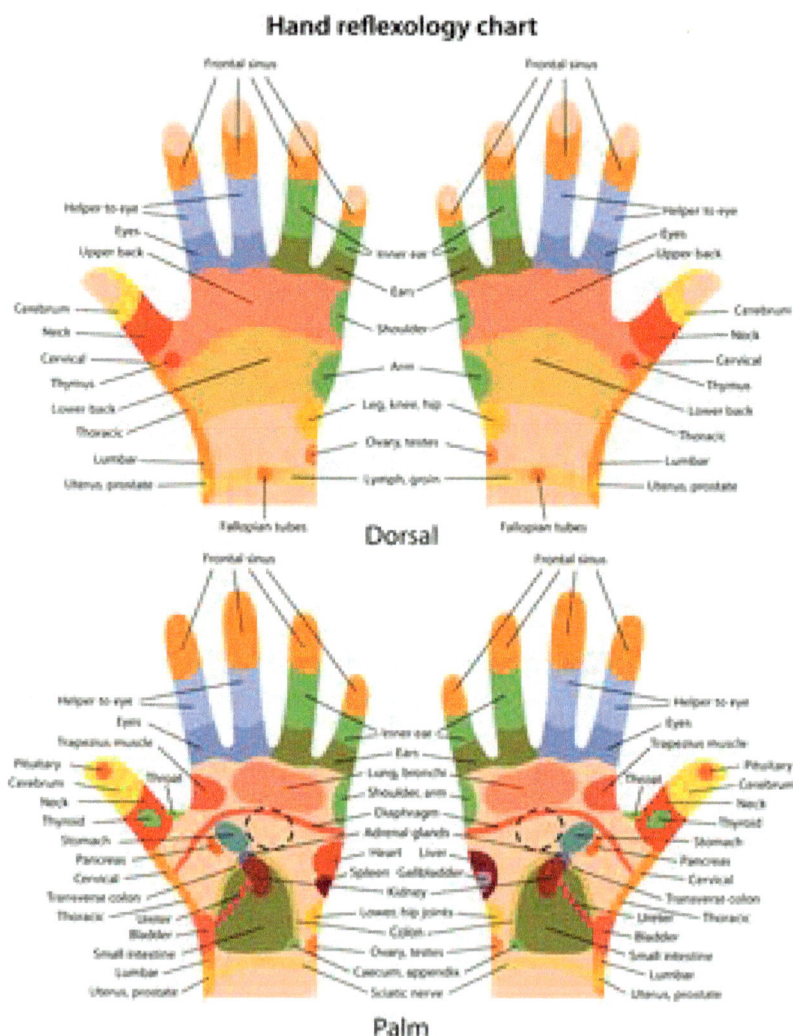

Hand Reflexology Chart

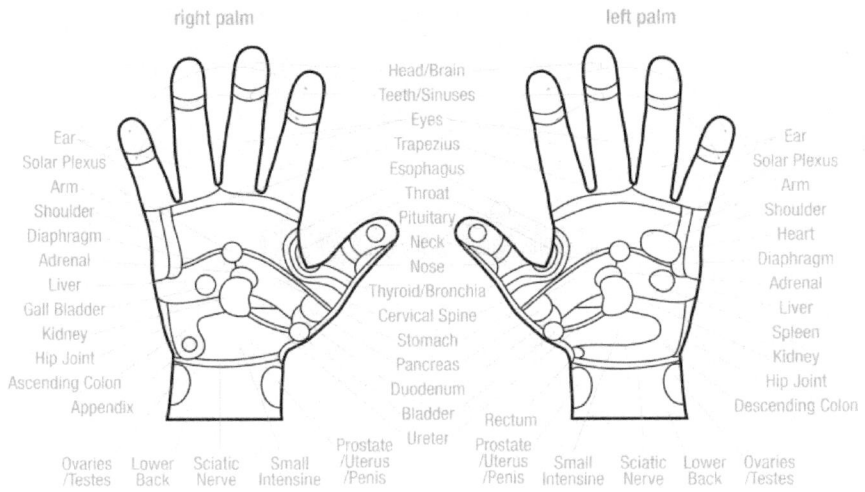

Just like your feet, hands also have reflex points for all your body organs and systems, as illustrated in the charts above. Hand reflexology works like feet reflexology, where pressure is applied to various parts of your hands, representing your body's major organs and systems, to initiate healing and relaxation.

Also, hand reflexology is quick and simple and can aid in alleviating various issues and ailments. The therapy has a reputation for providing instant relief from tension and pain.

Despite its simplicity, **the health benefits of hand reflexology can be classified into three main groups:**

- **Increased Flexibility:** Especially in seniors, hand reflexology can ease joint movement and improve mobility, such as in cases of rheumatoid arthritis.

- **Pain Relief:** This can range from pain relief associated with chronic ailments like osteoarthritis or cancer to everyday pain caused by repetitive motion.

- **Boost Circulation:** Poor blood circulation can occur owing to a variety of reasons such as an injury, long-term issues like blood clots, or Raynaud's, ailments which hand reflexology can help you to manage by easing their symptoms.

Additionally, hand reflexology can offer some form of relief for the following conditions:

- Irritable bowel syndrome

- Breathing problems and sinus

- Headaches

- Stress

- Symptoms of menopause

- Shoulder and back pain

Hand reflexology is just as effective as its foot counterpart while often remaining slightly more convenient. However, it is worth noting that ***the reflex points in your hands are a little deeper than those on your feet***. This means that for hand reflexology to be effective, the therapy usually requires more pressure than foot treatment.

Cross-Reflexes

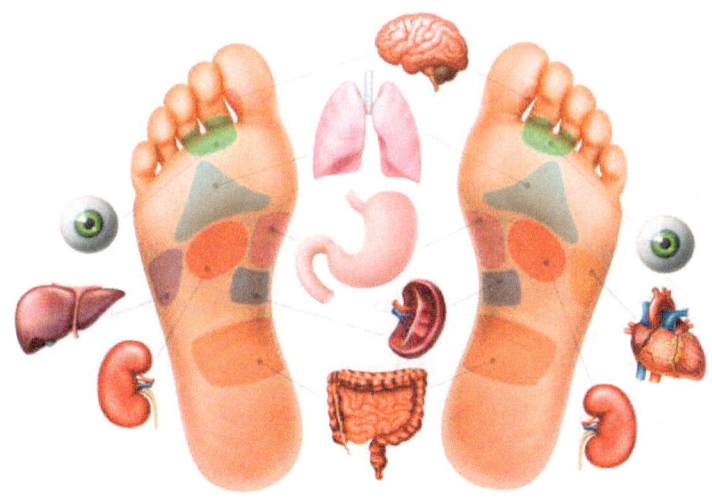

Suppose your feet are inaccessible for various reasons; for instance, you might be suffering from swelling, injury, a condition like gout, recuperating after foot surgery, or for any other reason. In that case, a cross-reflex approach can be applied. This concept originates from the zone therapy theory of **Dr. William Fitzgerald**.

We are equipped with energy zones that traverse the entire body length – from your toes, legs, head, fingers, arms, and head. According to this theory, the cross-reflexes that run up and down your body have a mirror effect. This means that therapy performed on your feet can affect the area around your arm or hand – and vice versa.

For example, if your ankle is sprained and swollen, it would not be possible for your reflexologist to work on your foot. The alternative would be to conduct reflexology on your wrist area to prevent more swelling, soreness, pain, or any other potential complication to your ankle. Or, if you have a broken leg, your reflexologist can work on the corresponding area in your arm to boost circulation on the injured leg and expedite the healing process as a result.

The cross-reflexes theory enables your reflexologist to treat parts of your body that would have otherwise been out-of-bounds. It also allows you to work on your own hands at your convenience or when issues arise suddenly, and you do not have immediate access to a reflexologist.

The principal cross-reflexes include:

- Fingers - toes
- Foot – hand
- The sole of the foot – palm of the hand
- Top of foot – palm of hand
- Ankle – wrist
- Calf – the inner area of the forearm
- Shin – outer section of the forearm
- Knee – elbow
- Thigh – upper arm
- Hip – shoulder

The cross-reflex theory shows that alternative options are available to your reflexologist if any part of your body is out of commission, preventing therapy from being administered directly. It helps to understand how your wrist can be used to reduce the swelling in your ankle or how the outer section of your forearm can hasten the healing of your fractured shin. Of course, the cross-flex theory also works the other way around – reflexology can be performed on your ankle to solve a wrist issue, and so on.

Let's move on to the next chapter to learn how to read and interpret feet in reflexology.

Chapter 4: Reading and Interpreting Feet in Reflexology

Your feet can provide a treasure trove of information to a reflexologist, especially concerning your state of health. To identify issues, your reflexologist, in most cases, will follow a few procedures to locate and identify reflex points that are out of balance or sensitive. Often, these reflexes correspond to specific parts of your body and signal the possibility of a problem in the respective area.

However, before any physical examination is carried out, the first phase is to **observe and evaluate your foot**. You may be surprised by how much information your feet can give about your general health, personality, and much more.

For example, if the skin on your feet is dry, it may indicate the presence of a hormonal imbalance or dehydration. The color of your feet is also crucial. Brightly colored feet could be a sign of hypertension, while cold, pale feet may signify poor blood circulation.

Simply put, the same way your feet carry you, they also carry the history of your life – through the pairs' color, texture, and structure.

Physical Examination

Your reflexologist identifies congested areas by **locating crystals** in your feet to pinpoint problematic areas. The crystals are made up of calcium or uric acid build-up in the nerve endings. For instance, if your lungs are not functioning correctly, God forbid, their regular muscular activity may slow down. As a result, the extremities of the organs' nerve endings are blocked.

Although this blockage might be minimal, it could be sufficient to reduce normal circulation to your lungs. Consequently, this denies the vital organs the ample supply of nutrients, oxygen, and blood they require to function while hampering your lung's ability to eject toxins.

When your reflexologist applies pressure to the crystals in your feet, they are broken up and dissolve into your bloodstream – rendering them harmless and unblocking the nerve endings of your lungs. Therefore, your reflexologist usually works on as many crystals as they are able to find or identifies the appropriate areas to conduct therapy according to your symptoms.

In addition, *if your reflexologist encounters a sensitive area on your feet during the therapy*, it could indicate the presence of a weakened area within your body. If the imbalance is corrected or treated with the use of reflexology immediately, a brewing condition or ailment may be averted before it strikes. Also, your reflexologist has to apply just the right pressure because too little or too much could lead to failure in tackling the underlying issue or, worse, provide a false reading.

Interestingly, reflexology is like a crystal ball – the therapy can detect current and past health issues that have probably been long forgotten. For example, if you had a hysterectomy 20 years ago, your reflexes will still be sensitive today. The reason? Your body remembers all your previous operations and injuries – the same way you do. It is also possible for your reflexologist to pick up a condition in your past that was resolved or suppressed, such as asthma, during your childhood.

In addition, reflex points in your hands and feet *can highlight areas of vulnerability or weakness, which can potentially cause future challenges*. This allows you to utilize reflexology as a preventative therapy and turn your attention to treatment, emotional well-being, lifestyle choices, and a healthy diet – to ensure you continue to enjoy good health.

Importance of Healthy Feet in Reflexology

Since your feet act as a crucial source of information in regard to your physical and emotional strengths and weaknesses, they need to be healthy to **avoid sending the wrong signals**. Another important role your feet play is to support your body weight; if your feet muscles weaken for whatever reason, it can have a negative effect on the tissue in your feet.

An abrupt change or impairment to any part of your body, including your feet, poses the risk of displacing your center of gravity. A good example is how a sedentary life can lead to knee, foot, and back problems with advancing age.

Your foot is made up of 20 muscles, 100 ligaments, a total of 26 bones, an intricate network of blood supply, and nerves. The bones are joined together by connective tissue, nerves, and blood vessels – under layers of skin. The two most essential functions of your feet are propulsion and weight-bearing, which require high levels of stability. Also, your feet must be flexible to adapt to rough and uneven surfaces. Any problems that may alter the structure of your feet could also affect your posture.

At the most basic level, reflexology can improve your feet's circulation. Poor posture, ill-fitting shoes, tension, and stress are some of the factors that may restrict blood flow to your feet, which can lead to a sluggish lymphatic and circulatory system. Such a scenario also means that contracting an infection, like a leg ulcer, may take an abnormally long period to heal.

When blood flow to your feet is wanting, it becomes difficult for white blood cells, oxygen-rich blood, and nutrients to access areas of your feet to fight infections and germs and remove toxins from your system. Therefore, regular reflexology ensures your feet remain healthy and boosts your body's circulation.

What Your Feet Reveal

As mentioned earlier, your feet can reveal your general state of health; more often than not, any issues present in your feet could be linked to issues in your body. How you choose to live your life, how you feel, your dietary habits and levels of activity or inactivity represent just a fraction of the information your reflexologist can learn courtesy of your feet.

For instance, limb feet might signal poor muscle tone, tense feet may point to a build-up of tension in your body, sweaty feet could be an indication that your hormone production system is on overdrive while swelling around your ankles may suggest a more serious problem that requires urgent medical attention.

Failure to look after your feet can also result in bunions, corns, ingrown toenails, hammertoes, calluses, heel pain, and other conditions that may affect your metabolism or posture. On the flip side, poor posture and metabolism could also contribute to these conditions, according to reflexologists.

Here are some of the most common foot conditions affecting approximately two-thirds of seniors to help you identify, prevent them, or seek help. Eradicating these conditions ensures your reflexology therapy is accurate, relaxing, and effective;

- **Bunions**

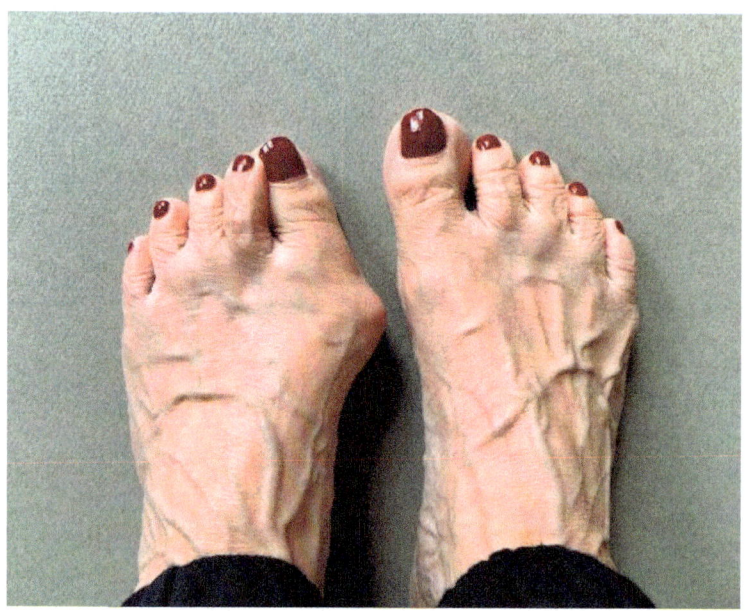

These appear as a thickened fluid-filled sac or bursa at the base of the big toe, which overlies the joint. Sometimes, a bunion may form on the fifth toe, making it feel inflamed or painful. Bunions are often caused by friction or persistent pressure emanating from an external agent, a joint injury or weakness, or foot displacement owing to the constant wearing of high-heeled, tight, or ill-fitting shoes. Bunions can also be a result of poor hygiene.

Bunions can be treated by wearing well-fitting shoes or using a protective pad for your feet to ease any discomfort you may experience. If all this fails, surgery can be a last resort.

- **Callous**

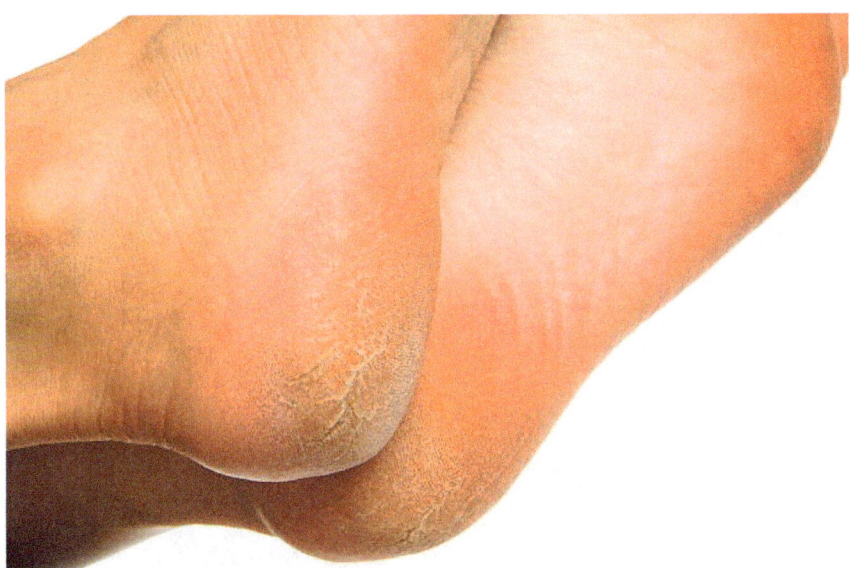

Callous describes an area that often appears on your big toe, tip of toes, ball of the foot, or on your heels, and the affected section looks like a thick hornlike skin, often discolored, dark-brown, or yellow. This is usually due to overbearing and persistent pressure on your foot, which normally occurs daily – and the condition can be painful.

In most cases, wearing ill-fitting shoes and standing or walking for extended periods are the main causes of this condition. You can easily treat callous by switching to well-fitting and comfortable shoes, adding a padded insole to your shoes, or carefully paring away the thickened area of your skin. Additionally, moisturizing your feet at least twice a day and using a pumice stone can eradicate the condition – but if any of these measures do not seem to work and symptoms persist, seek medical advice.

- **Corn**

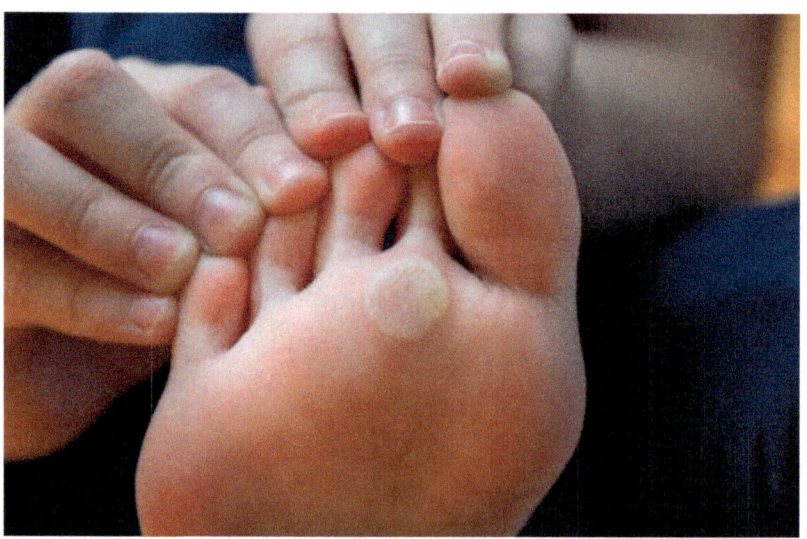

Corn is one of the most common problems found on feet. It is characterized by a cone-shaped, concentrated area of hard skin with no root. Often, the cone develops as a form of protection when your foot experiences excessive pressure or friction, which leads to your skin hardening and thickening.

There are two types of cones: **a hard one**, which usually appears on the top part of your toes or soles, and **a soft cone**, which, on the other hand, forms between your toes and, occasionally, underneath nails. However, both cones are caused by excessive friction and pressure and can be painful.

Wearing shoes designed with ample space for your toes is one way of preventing cones from developing. You can also apply small amounts of surgical spirit directly on the cones daily to help them dry up.

Alternatively, you can purchase a cone-removal adhesive that you simply place on top of your cone, and when you remove it a few days later, it also pulls out the corn with it. There are also creams that can eliminate it when applied to the cone. Alternatively, a Podiatrist can surgically remove a cone – especially if it is painful.

- **Ingrown Toenail**

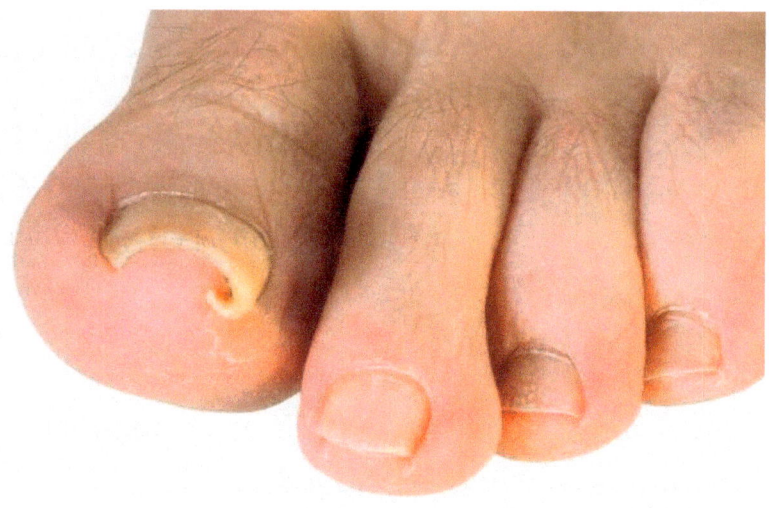

This is a painful condition in which one or both edges of your nail penetrate your big toe's adjacent skin and, as a result, become embedded in your skin's soft tissue. This may lead to bleeding, inflammation, and, ultimately, infection. This condition usually occurs when you trim your toenail along its side or cut it too short. Also, wearing shoes that are too tight and poor personal hygiene can cause ingrown toenails.

If possible, free the embedded toenail from the soft tissue by gently lifting or removing it using nail clippers. If the area on the side of your toe is swollen, apply a wet compress for a few minutes daily until the swelling goes down. Do not attempt to remove the toenail when swollen.

If the area is infected, it appears red, swollen, painful, and developing pus. In such a case, it would be best to have it surgically removed by a chiropodist.

These are just a few examples of foot conditions that need to be addressed, if present, before embarking on reflexology therapy. This ensures that these conditions do not mask any other issues you may have in the rest of your body and are ultimately missed by your reflexologist. Additionally, healthy feet reduce the risk of a false reading and interpretation during reflexology – and a pair of healthy feet also contributes to your overall well-being.

What Your Nails Reveal in Reflexology

Interestingly, the nails on your feet and hands tend to grow faster when your hormone levels fluctuate. Nails grow at a rate of 3mm (an eighth of an inch) every month. But their growth can be slowed considerably or stopped altogether in case of ill health.

Often, if you cut your nails, or for some unexplained reason, they stop growing and then resume growth. A line that runs across your nail appears, referred to as Beau's line, which is caused by the interruption in the protein formation of your nail plate.

Nails are made of keratin, a fibrous protein also found in your hair. Consequently, it is common for seniors experiencing hair loss (alopecia) to have thin nails or find their nails dropping off altogether. But when your nails are shiny, flexible, and healthy, the water and molecules between the keratin layers are largely responsible for this.

What Are You Eating?

In reflexology, your nails have the ability to reveal your dietary habits and your current health status through the following pointers:

- ***If your nails appear cracked***, it could be an indication that you are dehydrated and you need to increase your water intake

- ***Brittle and dry nails*** can be a sign that your body may have a deficiency of calcium and vitamin A. Oily fish like pilchards or sardines, eggs, cheese, and liver are some examples of rich sources of vitamin A, while cheese, purple sprouting broccoli, canned salmon, milk sardines, and yogurt can replenish calcium in your body.

- ***Curved nail ends,*** which are too rounded and exhibit excessive dryness, may suggest a lack of vitamin B12 in your body. Usually, vegans are at a higher risk since the only source of vitamin B12 comes from animal products – eggs, fish, and meat.

- ***A pale nail bed*** may be a sign of anemia. This is a condition where your blood does not have sufficient amounts of healthy red blood cells – the most common cause is a lack of iron in your body. To correct this deficiency, include foods like leafy green vegetables, lean meat, dried apricots, sardines, oily fish, and liver in your diet.

- ***Concave, spoon-shaped, or nails with ridges*** could be symptoms of a disorder known as koilonychia – another iron deficiency. Your doctor can establish if the condition is present through a simple hemoglobin test, and you can increase your intake of the same rich-iron foods as those for anemia mentioned in the previous point.

Basic Nail Care

The aging process changes every part of your body – finger and toenails included. By now, you probably have noticed that your nails may have become harder, thicker, brittle in texture, duller in color, and take longer to grow. In addition to these changes, you are more susceptible to developing fungal infections close to or on your nail bed.

This probability becomes common, especially since you are always advised to wear socks and shoes indoors to reduce the risk of falls, keep your feet warm, and protect them. But there's a setback in this arrangement. When your feet are cooped up in shoes and socks most of the time, the resultant warm and damp conditions create the perfect environment for fungus to grow, spread, and flourish.

This emphasizes the importance of taking care of your nails to avoid potential problems and boost your level of comfort, which will make a huge contribution to your overall quality of life. It also ensures your reflexology sessions are effective and provide an accurate picture of your health status during sessions.

This can be achieved by simply paying more attention to your nail care routine by implementing the following grooming strategies:

- ***When cutting nails, choose your preferred tool for the job carefully.*** Either use custom-made scissors for nails or fingernail clippers. Clean your tool frequently because it can collect dirt and bacteria. You can use alcohol to disinfect it, followed by a thorough cleaning using hot water; dry your tool completely before safely storing it.

- ***Always cut nails straight across or perpendicularly.*** Trimming your nails in a curved pattern is a leading cause of ingrown nails. Also, use a nail file or emery board to smoothen the edges of your nails to prevent rough edges from inflicting damage to your skin, which is thinner.

- ***Do not cut off, push back, or pull out cuticles*** – leave them alone. Cuticles act as protection from damage to your nail bed. The opening left after removing your cuticles tends to form pathways for pathogens and bacteria to access your skin, which significantly increases your risk of infection or illness.

Chapter 5: How A Reflexology Session Looks Like and What to Expect

When you are not sure of what to expect during your first reflexology session, you might feel apprehensive and probably a little nervous – which need not be the case.

A professional reflexologist can conduct therapy in a clinic or at their home or operate a mobile practice capable of moving to wherever you are. The sessions can be performed using a massage table or a reclining chair. In the event you are experiencing mobility issues, having a therapist visit your home is usually the best option. This is because you will receive the treatment in a comfortable environment, you will not aggravate your mobility issues any further, and immediately after the session, you can relax – instead of expending yourself commuting back home.

If you choose to visit a clinic or the home of your reflexologist, they will probably have a massage table or reclining chair available. However, if neither of these two pieces of furniture is available at your home, therapy can still be carried out in your bed, an armchair, a sofa, or a simple garden chair.

Place two pillows to support your head for comfort and enable your therapist to observe your facial expression during the session if you choose to conduct the session in bed. During reflexology, eye contact is important; it enables your practitioner to identify sore reflex points through your facial reaction. Place another pillow under your knees to provide support to your lower back and another two pillows under your feet to ensure they are at a height that is comfortable for your reflexologist to work.

When using a garden chair, armchair, or sofa, you can place pillows under your feet and a low stool on the floor to elevate your feet to the right level, comfortably within reach for your therapist.

Personal Preps

To ensure you get the most out of reflexology, you also need to make some preparations on a personal level. The following tips should enable you to reap maximum benefits from your therapy:

- **Relax Your Mind and Body:** Ensure you feel comfortable, unrushed, and settled before your session. Immediately before and after therapy, avoid scheduling any strenuous activities. If possible, observe a grace period to enjoy a moment of relaxation – before and after your session.

- **Wear Comfortable Clothing:** Your reflexologist only needs to work on your feet or hands to access their reflex maps. But since your session will also be relaxing, it would be wise to wear loose, comfortable clothing complemented by everyday footwear. If you can, avoid wearing jewelry, a watch, or other fashion accessories.

- **Diet:** Preferably, do not overeat or begin your session when hungry – eat just the right amount. In case you have sugar issues, you can always have a small protein snack immediately before your therapy begins. Some reflexologists also offer a snack on request, that is, if your session is scheduled to be held in a clinic.

- **Hydration:** Since reflexology encourages your body to eject toxins from its system, you will probably feel thirsty during and after your session is over. When your body is well hydrated, it responds better to therapy. Therefore, ensure you are hydrated before your session begins.

- **Stimulants and Therapy:** Energy drinks, coffee, black or green tea, and chocolate drinks should be avoided at least two hours before and after your reflexology session. The caffeine and theobromine (the chemical found in chocolate and similar to caffeine) in these drinks are stimulants that affect your nervous system and can counteract the positive effects of reflexology.

- **Alcohol:** When reflexology and alcohol come together, reports have shown that it results in negative effects. When the numbing effect of alcohol and the stimulating effect of therapy combine, it prevents you from being in touch with your body. As a result, it becomes difficult for your therapist to judge the right amount of pressure to apply on your foot to ensure your reflex points are sufficiently invigorated in order to trigger healing. Therefore, it is a good idea to avoid alcohol at least 24 hours before – and after therapy.

- **Health Self-Assessment:** In case you experience sudden symptoms, such as a skin rash or sore throat, that could indicate a contagious illness, it is crucial to resolve them before your in-person session to avoid spreading infections around unwittingly.

- **Stay Away From Distractions:** Switch off your phone and TV (if therapy is conducted at home), and avoid any other distractions capable of stealing your attention in the course of your session. Try to direct your full attention to your body and the ongoing therapy. However, chatting with your therapist as they work on you is okay.

Also, it helps to have knowledge of your health history and be informed about the reflexology goals you intend to accomplish as well. This information can assist your therapist in drawing up a session plan to guide them on areas that may require special emphasis or care during therapy.

Setting the Right Mood

Depending on where your session is conducted, most therapists set the scene to ensure they create a relaxed, comfortable, and 'healing' environment – which also boosts your confidence. Some of the additions that may be present in your session during your visit to a clinic or reflexologist home could include, but are not limited to:

- **Scents:** Your therapist may opt to light a scented candle or burn essential oils before your arrival to promote a relaxed ambiance. However, most always ensure the fragrance left in the air is not too heavy to avoid aggravating your senses, triggering a respiratory condition, or allergic response.

- **Music:** Soft music is both soothing and relaxing. It is common for reflexologists to play soft music in the background to enable you to relax and enjoy the session. In fact, music has been [shown to reduce](https://pubmed.ncbi.nlm.nih.gov/34955298/)[9] anxiety and pain and increase the quality of your sleep when played during massage and reflexology sessions, according to studies.

- **Lighting:** During reflexology, your therapist may also dim the lights to create a relaxing ambiance. Some reflexologists prefer to switch off overhead lights that directly shine in your eyes and turn on floor lights instead.

- **Water:** A glass or bottle of water should be readily available at your side and within easy reach during your session. As mentioned earlier, water aids your body in flushing out the toxins released during therapy, and taking sips of water between your sessions can help the process. Besides, after your session, you will likely feel parched.

---

[9] https://pubmed.ncbi.nlm.nih.gov/34955298/

The Main Event

Typically, a reflexology session can **last anywhere between 30 to 90 minutes** on average. Before the session begins, your reflexologist will conduct a brief history health check to ensure your needs and current health status align with the therapy. You may inquire about what you expect to gain from your session(s).

Next, your reflexologist will give you a brief rundown of how the therapy works. Remember that the therapy's objective is not to cure any ailments and should not be considered a substitute for medical treatment. Sometimes, you may be requested to sign a consent form – although this is not standard practice; in other places, a consent form may not be featured anywhere.

If you have any questions you need to ask or concerns to air, this is usually the best time to make your voice heard – and the answers provided should be to your satisfaction. Also, if you feel your reflexologist is evasive, not forthcoming, or dismissive in their responses, or if you no longer feel comfortable continuing with your session, this would be the perfect moment to opt out and cancel your appointment.

After an evaluation of your health needs, ***your reflexologist will decide whether to work on your feet, hands, or both***. For feet reflexology, you may be asked to sit or lie down and remove your shoes and socks only. Your feet will be washed and soaked in warm water for a few minutes to sanitize and relax the muscles in your feet, which makes it easier for your therapist to access your reflex points. Your reflexologist will then dry your feet and hold them at chest level.

Your therapist will then proceed to visually assess your feet for rashes, bunions, open wounds, warts, or any other issues that could have an impact on reflexology. They may also inquire about any leg or foot pain or injury that can stand in the way of therapy. Your reflexologist will then begin to work on your feet.

Regardless of your health issues or condition, your reflexologist will give you the entire pattern of therapy – beginning from your toes and working their way down to your heels. During the session, your practitioner may use several techniques to extend the necessary pressure to all the reflex points on your feet.

A common practice is to start by activating the reflexes corresponding to one side of your body, then move on to the next until your whole body is covered. This approach addresses muscle groups, internal organs, nerves, bones, and glands. If you have a specific issue, such as a migraine or heartburn, your reflexologist will gently feel the corresponding point and work on it. But they will also work on all areas of your foot by applying gentle pressure. This unblocks any congestion and stimulates nerve pathways, which, in turn, facilitates the relaxation response of your entire body.

An important point to understand is that reflexology invigorates your nervous system to carry out the job of balancing and releasing. The main objective is to bring your entire body into balance – which then causes pain to subside. When your reflexologist finds congestion, tightness, or pain, the pressure they apply on the area in question is supposed to bring your body back into balance.

Later, your therapist may return to that specific spot towards the end of your session to ensure the pain or congestion was successfully released. Throughout the session, your reflexologist will stay present, calm, grounded, and in a centered state of awareness.

Most practitioners have a calming and peaceful routine to close the session, which may involve stroking your foot or hand in a certain way. This is also to ensure you feel nurtured and comforted.

Once the session is over, take your time to bring yourself back to the present moment as you enjoy your relaxed state. Your therapist may suggest that you hydrate with water as you rest for a while. When you feel comfortable enough, you can grab your belongings and leave.

Note: Pay close attention to your body for the next few hours and the signals it sends. In case something unexpected comes up, your reflexologist should always be easily accessible – preferably on the phone.

Follow-up Sessions

Scheduling subsequent reflexology sessions depends on your health status and the reason behind seeking therapy. However, it is essential to note that reflexology outcomes are usually subtle and cumulative. This means your likelihood of reaping maximum benefits increases with regular sessions. For example, conducting one session a week for the next eight weeks tends to be more effective than having one session every three months. But, you may require more frequent sessions if you are battling a certain condition or illness.

For instance, you can have one reflexology session every week for the next 6 to 8 weeks and one *'tune-up'* session every four weeks after that.

How Should You Expect to Feel After a Reflexology Session?

Your first reflexology experience may vary, ranging from a general feeling of relaxation, tingling, or a sense of *'lightness,'* warmth, to a feeling of energy moving through your body. This may also include a sense of heightened communication between every nerve, valve, organ, gland, and muscle in your body.

Other common physical and emotional responses after your first reflexology session may comprise some of the following reactions, which are normal:

- Feeling light-headed

- The disappearance of all discomfort and pain

- Thirst

- Sighing deeply

- Perspiration of your feet and hands

- Feeling hot

- Feeling slightly chilled or cold

- An overwhelming desire to sleep

- Relaxed, loose muscles and organs

- Contraction of muscle groups – which is rare

- Coughing

- Laughing

- Crying

- Frequent bowel movements, skin rashes, or pimples due to the elimination of toxins

- Increased energy levels

- A significant surge in the number of mobile joints

Normally, the reactions after a reflexology session are subtle, and most seniors do not associate them with therapy. A huge chunk of the reactions are positive indications, showing reflexology activates the healing process. On the other hand, other symptoms can be linked to your body's attempt to revert to a state of harmony and balance – most reactions vanish after 24-48 hours.

The Healing Crisis Reaction

Reflexology boosts your body's ability to heal, and you should expect some response. Typically, most seniors experience sensations of feeling rejuvenated, deeply relaxed, energized, and overall well-being. However, occasionally, reflexology can lead to a healing crisis reaction. When this happens, your symptoms may be amplified before you feel better.

Interpret this as a cleansing process where your body is getting rid of existing toxins – it could be the much-needed turning point in the pattern of your condition. If you have a lot of impurities in your system or are going through an emotional phase in your life, chances of experiencing a healing crisis reaction increase considerably.

However, this should not be cause for concern because the intense symptoms or reactions **tend to pass within 24 hours**. Drinking around 2 liters of water a day prior to your session, on the day of your appointment, and the day after treatment can go a long way in easing your body's response. This is because water helps flush out toxins out of your body while, at the same time, taming the intensity of the healing crisis reaction.

Try to steer clear of stimulating drinks, such as alcohol, tea, or coffee, during these few days. This is because they can diminish the effectiveness of your reflexology session.

Your first session is also expected to be a little painful in some areas, especially if you are experiencing a condition or illness. Your reflexologist may reduce the pressure applied to your sensitive reflex points to avoid discomfort and ensure your therapy is more bearable.

Unusual chilliness, sudden sweating, feelings of distress, faintness, and nausea are less common and referred to as hypersensitive responses. In case they prove too intense during a session, your reflexologist can allow a pause and a drink of water to ease the response.

However, in most maiden sessions, most seniors respond well to therapy and appreciate reflexology's positive impact on their health and emotional well-being.

Chapter 6: Emotional and Mental Health Implications of Reflexology

Apart from managing pain and aches associated with aging or chronic illness, reflexology also has the ability to make significant contributions to your emotional and mental health. Mental and physical health are inter-reliant – deprived physical well-being can lead to emotional distress, and you may eventually develop mental health problems and vice versa.

For example, when physical health declines, it can translate to a loss of independence or the necessity to adapt to a totally new environment – scenarios that can affect your mental health in diverse ways.

Some of **the common triggers of mental health conditions** may include:

- Loss and grief

- Increased social isolation

- Illness

- An abrupt shift in living arrangements

- Frailty and loss of independence

- Financial stress

On the other hand, mental health conditions have an adverse effect on physical health. If you are not doing well emotionally and mentally, this can negatively affect your immunity. This, in turn, makes you prone to diseases, healing takes longer, and treating chronic illnesses becomes more complicated, among several other potential challenges.

Physical illnesses and conditions that usually affect seniors and are known to contribute to mental health problems include:

- Obesity

- Cognitive decline

- High blood pressure

- Heart disease

- Alzheimer's

- Weak immune system

Sadly, mental health issues bedeviling seniors are often overlooked, unnoticed, unidentified, or dismissed as *'normal'* occurrences that come with aging, which is not entirely true. There is also the stigma that surrounds attempting to access mental health care, which creates hurdles for seniors, as it leads to reluctance to seek help.

According to WHO statistics[10], 14% of seniors aged 60 and above live with a mental condition – which is a ratio of around one in four senior citizens. Yet, very few seek medical intervention. The mental needs of seniors are unique, and the common issues that affect seniors over 60 include:

- Anxiety

- Dementia

- Depression

- Suicide

- Substance abuse

- Frequent mental distress (FMS)

---

[10] https://cdn.who.int/media/docs/default-source/gho-documents/global-health-estimates/ghe2019

Among seniors over 60s, dementia and depression are the most prevalent, with anxiety following closely. Also, when compared to other age groups, the [highest rate][11] of suicide is witnessed in older adults. Apparently, seniors aged 85 years and above happen to have the highest suicide rate, while the 75-84 age group takes second position. Some of the major contributing factors are loneliness and social isolation.

Although loneliness and isolation may sound identical, they are not necessarily similar. For example, you may live alone but enjoy an active social life and a strong relationship with your family. On the flip side, you can feel extremely lonely, yet friends and family always surround you. Since we are naturally wired to be social beings, the inability to connect with others or lose your sense of community can change your perception of the world – which may have a negative impact on your mental health as well.

Additionally, at this phase of your life, your mental health is not only shaped by social and physical environments. The cumulative influences of your earlier life experiences and specific stressors in regard to aging could also have a major impact. Potential loss of your intrinsic capacity, decline in

---

[11] https://www.webmd.com/mental-health/recognizing-suicidal-behavior

your functional ability, and exposure to any form of adversity are all factors that can result in psychological distress.

It is during times like these that reflexology can change your life.

A Case in Point

Hilda was overjoyed to retire at 65 from her career as an investment consultant for a leading bank – a job she had held for over 40 years. Her retirement was planned well in advance. She wanted to spend more time with her family – her husband, son, and daughter, who were in their late and early twenties, respectively. Hilda had also planned to direct her energies to a farm they had purchased with her husband of 35 years, John.

Two years after her retirement, all her plans were in disarray. John was diagnosed with cancer, which was advanced. A year later, he passed on. Her son, who was in the army, was posted to a foreign country, and her daughter was employed by a firm that was based in a faraway city – and just like that, Hilda was all alone. A situation she had not anticipated, planned, or prepared for.

Although her son and daughter kept in touch regularly, physical meetings were rare – about once a year. Feelings of loneliness coupled with stress started gradually creeping in. Soon, the impact became evident when her health began to fail, and the loneliness she felt only made matters worse.

Just when Hilda was about to hit rock bottom, she was introduced to reflexology by a concerned friend, and the therapy turned her life around. It gifted her new awareness by providing an outlet for her stress and an avenue to rejuvenate and find balance. She then found meaning and a new purpose to live.

Soon, Hilda's health took a U-turn, and within a year, she was back to her healthy old self again and going about the activities she loved and enjoyed with renewed vigor and enthusiasm. In addition to the medical treatment she received for her physical ailments, Hilda also embraced reflexology as alternative care, and this combination worked wonders – the outcome was a holistic approach to healing.

How Does Reflexology Boost Emotional and Mental Health?

- **Combating Emotional Pain**

Your body reacts to negative nerve stimulation through physical or emotional pain. But when you receive positive strategic stimulation (read reflexology), your body increases its production of endorphins – your feel-good hormones.

Apart from creating a buffer between your emotional health and disease, this reaction also acts as a catalyst to help reverse the negative effects. According to a published study[12], 80% of the development of any ailment is contributed by stress/anxiety/depression. The same study also discovered that as a response to reflexology, your body releases your body's pain-relieving chemical, endorphins, which guide your body on the most effective way to adapt to any damage inflicted – physical, emotional, or mental.

When reflexology triggers the production of endorphins, your body develops resilience against negative emotional effects.

- **Tackling Stress, Depression, and Anxiety Symptoms**

Currently, mental health issues, especially among seniors, have reached epidemic levels. According to the National Institute of Mental Health[13], major depression ranks top as the most common mental health disorder. The condition is a type of mood disorder characterized by immense suffering and distress. Additionally, depression can lead to physical, mental, and social functioning impairments and is capable of

---

[12] https://www.ncbi.nlm.nih.gov/pmc/articles/PMC4624523/
[13] https://www.nimh.nih.gov/health/statistics/prevalence/major-depression-among-adults.shtml

adversely affecting the course and treatment of other chronic illnesses.

Although the rate of depression tends to increase with age, contrary to popular belief, the condition is not a normal part of aging. Unfortunately, depression in seniors[14] is often under-recognized, left untreated, and under-treated, which compounds the problem even further.

However, it is well-known that depression, anxiety, and stress are linked to chemical imbalances in your brain, poor nutrition, sleep deprivation, pain or disability, genetics, decreased blood flow to major organs, and negative thinking, among numerous other potential factors. You are also probably aware that a quick-fix solution does not exist. But in your arsenal, reflexology is one weapon among several others you can effectively utilize in conjunction with modern medicine to regain and improve your mental health.

A powerful way reflexology boosts your mental and emotional health is by enhancing blood circulation in your body, which, in turn, ensures crucial nutrients and oxygen are consistently supplied to your brain, injecting vitality into your body's systems and mental faculties.

---

[14] http://www.surgeongeneral.gov/library/mentalhealth/chapter5/sec1.html

- **Relaxation Effect**

Arguably, the most active and overworked part of your body happens to be your feet. While a reflexology session can provide much-needed respite to your feet by relieving any tension build-up, this process is also directly connected to your emotional and mental well-being. During such moments, you gain mental clarity in the form of new great ideas or even solutions to problems that have bothered you for some time. Reflexology's ability to rest your body and revitalize your emotions begins by simply relaxing your muscles.

Reflexology enables improved relaxation by easing the pain and aches in your joints, improving circulation, and unblocking clogged nerve endings. As a result, anxiety, stress, and depression are reduced, promoting healthy sleeping habits and overall mental wellness. These traits make reflexology an ideal tool to prevent cognitive deterioration and diseases; in the process, your moods are uplifted as a bonus.

When your sleep pattern is improved, common incidents of dozing off during the day become a thing of the past. This frees up more time for activities that you enjoy. This stimulation of your mental and emotional faculties serves as fuel to develop sharper cognitive abilities, which prevents and curbs the symptoms of debilitating conditions such as Alzheimer's.

- **The Magic Behind Human Touch**

From infancy to old age, the need for human touch is a basic need. This seemingly small and irrelevant action enables you to feel a deep physical and emotional connection. Without touch, it is common to feel isolated, lonely, and unwanted – a recipe for mental and emotional issues. Reflexology is a hands-on and connective therapy that positively impacts your mental health.

Research studies[15] have shown that touch calms your nervous system and slows your heartbeat. Human touch also has the ability to lower your blood pressure and the production of cortisol – your stress hormone. Touch also triggers the release of a hormone known as oxytocin that promotes emotional bonding with other people.

---

[15] https://www.jstor.org/stable/986002

[Another study](#)[16] that used a PET scan showed that your brain quietens in response to stress when a person holds your hand. The greatest effect was recorded when the handheld belonged to a loved one, but the effect is still present even if a stranger is involved.

The positive impact of human touch in the study also extended to the response of your body's immune system. It was discovered that people deprived of human touch were more likely to suffer from diseases of the immune system. This is the crucial therapeutic benefit of human touch that reflexology offers you and your mental health.

- **Handling Effects of Medication**

It is common, as you age, to find that you are taking prescription drugs for one reason or another. But over the years, how your body processes medicine changes, and you become increasingly prone to a variety of side effects that may include muscle weakness, nausea, loss of sleep, or even dizziness. Other side effects you may experience include

---
[16]

https://www.tandfonline.com/doi/abs/10.1080/1525024.2011.572046

delirium, confusion, and a dip in moods, which could also cause mental distress.

Reflexology can reduce the side effects of medication your doctor may have prescribed. When pressure is applied to your reflex points during a session, it changes the messages associated with side effects that your nerves send to your brain. This reduces the intensity of any side effects you may be experiencing related to prescription medicine. The relaxing effect of the therapy also plays a huge role in reducing side effects.

Apart from aiding a quick recovery, therapy also alleviates the physical and mental strain of enduring uncomfortable side effects.

- **Improving Brain Power**

Mental health conditions have one thing in common. They all originate from a single source – your brain. Reflexology, as we have already established, stimulates your nerve endings and opens up your neural pathways. As a result, information to your brain is much faster and more effective. Consequently, the speed at which your brain processes this information increases, and so does your physical and cognitive response times. Your memory, focus, and sharpness also receive a major boost.

- **Providing Convalescence Relief**

Receiving bad news about your health can be a stress-filled event; regardless of your resilience, keeping things straight will still be difficult. Your stress and anxiety levels can also increase if you are due to undergo surgery. When this happens, all your focus will most probably be directed towards your physical health – and your mental health is sidelined in the process.

But for your health to bounce back and fully recover, it is important to strike a balance between your ability to cope with post-surgical stress and address your mental health at the same time. Whatever circumstances may have led you down the path of surgery, it could also mean that you may have been dealing with health issues for quite a while, which also negatively impacts your mental health.

The constant clinic visits and medical bills will also take a toll on your emotional health. This makes it difficult to draw a line between post-surgical and recovery stress. Interestingly, even after a successful surgical procedure, including positive signs that indicate achieving a full recovery, negative emotions, such as feelings of hopelessness, can still be present.

A combination of seeking support from your doctor, family, and friends and signing up for reflexology sessions can be the winning formula to combat post-surgical and recovery stress. Adopting this strategy can also facilitate a faster healing process and create the positive attitude necessary for recovery.

Parting Shot

Although reflexology has been with us for over five centuries, it was not until recently that the therapy's true significance as a form of complementary therapy was fully appreciated.

Kindly note that there is a big difference between alternative and complementary therapies. Alternative therapies are offered to replace standard treatments, while complementary therapies are offered alongside standard treatments. Reflexology falls under this category of therapies that work in harmony with others.

While modern medicine has achieved groundbreaking breakthroughs that were previously thought impossible, practices like reflexology, yoga, acupuncture, and mindfulness can create inroads into areas that contemporary medical procedures and drugs have not managed to cover adequately. But when modern medicine and complementary forms of therapy combine forces, they become indomitable, and diseases suddenly become the prey – to your advantage.

When faced with a challenge, you typically throw all your resources, time, energy, and even mind power to overcome it.

Sometimes, you are unsure whether your strategy will work to deal with the challenge, but you do it all the same.

The same strategy should apply to any physical or mental health issues you may encounter as the years go by – and reflexology is one option that works well with other forms of treatment. Unlike life's challenges, where you are not sure whether your intended approach will produce the desired results, evidence shows that reflexology is effective in helping to reduce the symptoms associated with numerous physical and mental health conditions to a large extent.

The pain, discomfort, and stress accompanying any illness can significantly impact your recovery time and determine how an ailment affects you. But if you can ease the stress, pain, and discomfort through reflexology, more than half the battle is already won, making it easier to manage your condition. Also, the psychological benefits of the therapy, which include boosting feelings of overall well-being, are priceless when it comes to combatting any ailment.

Apparently, your foot hosts a total of 7,000 nerve endings connected to the rest of your body parts, organs, and systems, making your feet a central and ideal gateway to all the other areas of your body. Also, on a daily basis, your feet bear the weight of roughly 1,000 tons, and reflexology eases some of the punishment your feet have to take.

The pressure applied to your feet's reflex points to stimulate healing is minimal, meaning no pain, no prescription drugs are administered, and the therapy is effective for several health conditions. Additionally, gains range from improved blood circulation, reduced stress, improved mobility, and relaxation to the cultivation of a sense of well-being.

This means reflexology is generally safe for seniors and has far-reaching benefits. There are approximately 17 million practitioners worldwide, which shows the exponential growth the therapy has witnessed over the years. It also means you will not need to look very far in search of a trained reflexologist, which is convenient.

Another huge advantage of reflexology is its rare ability to provide holistic therapy. Most therapies in the same class offer therapy to specific areas, systems, or parts of your body. But no system, organ, or part of your body is out of reach or inaccessible for reflexology – a feat no other therapy or treatment can match.

As technology continues to evolve, its long tentacles are bound to extend to reflexology. Already, there is talk about applications that can assist your reflexologist in monitoring your progress and enable you to provide regular feedback to your therapist – a welcome addition set to improve the practice.

Although reflexology has proved beneficial to your physical and mental health, it still **requires the support of other practices,** such as observing a healthy lifestyle, ultimately enabling you to enjoy the therapy's maximum benefits. Also, exercise due diligence when booking a reflexology session to ensure your therapist is well-trained, qualified, and licensed to practice by relevant regulatory bodies.

All seniors should enjoy the benefits of reflexology. If you are unsure whether you qualify for therapy, consulting your doctor first would be the best way to find out. Any therapy with the potential to deliver less pain, quality of life improvement, reduced stress, uplifted mood, no side effects, peace of mind, and a sense of overall well-being is definitely worth a shot – all things considered.

PS: I'd like your feedback. If you are happy with this book, please leave a review on Amazon.

Please leave a review for this book on Amazon by visiting the page below:

https://amzn.to/2VMR5qr

Printed in Dunstable, United Kingdom

66273020R00057